GOD'S ELECT LADIES

Sabrina P. Evans

GOD'S ELECT LADIES

by

Sabrina P. Evans

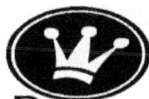

LOWBAR
PUBLISHING COMPANY

905 South Douglas Avenue • Nashville, Tennessee 37204
Phone: 615-972-2842
E-mail: Lowbarpublishingcompany@gmail.com
Web site: www.Lowbarbookstore.com

Lowbar Publishing Company 905 S. Douglas Ave.
Nashville, Tennessee 37204
615-972-2842
Lowbarpublishingcompany@gmail.com
www.Lowbarbookstore.com

Editor: Tracy
Graphic and Cover Design Artist: Aalishaa

Printed in the United States of America
ISBN: 13: 978-1-7329202-2-4
For additional information or to contact the author for workshops or seminars, please email the author at evang8sabrina@gmail.com or Lowbar Publishing Company.

TABLE OF CONTENTS

Dedication

GOD'S ELECT LADIES

In memory of my mother, Mary T. Walton, and the many women who carry the survival torch every day, reminding us that our strength is in Him who created us in His image, God our Father, Jesus our Lord, and the Holy Spirit our Helper!

Introduction

Women of Strength, Passion, and Faith

Thank you for choosing God's Elect Ladies, a book that allows you to share the journey of some remarkable women. Women of great courage and fervor, true survivors who continue to press through everyday challenges with diagnoses of various infirmities. You will gain knowledge and insight from the information gathered about different diseases and some personal consequences these diseases have on women in their individual lives. Although you may identify with some of these ailments, our prayer is that you find strength in your time of weakness to rely upon your faith moving forward. As I thought over various illnesses and how they have touched some family and friends of mine, it seemed as if my spirit could hear the cries of some asking the question: "Lord why me?" Perhaps a number of you are wondering, "What have I done to deserve this affliction, or my child, mother, sibling, or spouse, this sickness, disease, or whatever the condition may be?" I know all too well. Will the pages of this book hold your answers? For some of you, hopefully, it will but for others maybe not. No one can claim to know or understand the mind of God, "it is He that has made us and not we ourselves," or to be more specific, we are his chosen vessels, why our Father would allow anyone to face sickness seems to defy common understanding. However, we can rest assured that He is with us. Is it possible to find purpose in our suffering? Yes, I strongly believe so. What we know and believe is, God uses our struggles to His glory as greatly referenced in the scriptures. He permissively allows sickness. Yes, nothing can happen unless the Almighty permits it. He sees and knows everything. His plan for each of us and His thoughts toward us are of peace, good and not evil. In the Bible, we read how Satan, our adversary, afflicted Job. Job is someone about whom the scripture states that he loved and trusted God. However, God allowed it. This is a very interesting or rather mind-boggling story of someone who lost all: children, livestock, servants, etc. and yet, he worshipped God in truth and spirit, refusing to allow his devastating circumstances to stagger and dampen his faith in the Lord. "Why would Job maintain his faith in God?" you may ask. It is because the fight is not ours but the Lord's. Satan hates the faith we have in our Creator, but Jesus has given us victory. Therefore, Job's story has a great ending in spite of the horrendous circumstances. There are many scriptures that supports our Father's love. Psalms 103:3 declares that the Lord forgives our sins and heals all our diseases. But how do we see healing? Do we see it as a miracle, a process, no more pain and suffering or death? Acknowledging this truth can be difficult; life doesn't always give us the results we desire. One of the most un-talked about fruits of the spirit in Galatians 5:22 is longsuffering. How long is long? What is the lesson to be learned? Is there a purpose for what I am going through? My answer to that is, there is absolutely a purpose. Considering we all are different, I submit there are various levels of healing and documentation to support them. One other thing to consider is that God can consent to certain experiences in the lives of His people to give testimony of His greatness as well as their level of faith. Healing reveals itself in a broader perspective than just the physical. Healing takes upon the notions of strength and character. Healing can be seen in mental stability, emotional balance, and spiritual ease or rest. These assessments require a commitment to an authentic bond with God and us. Often, the hesitance to forgive prolongs and intensifies sickness and pain. Let me pause here because we are usually wont to blame something or someone for our illnesses and travails. In periods of plight, we often become angry with God, others and ourselves. We harbor un-forgiveness. And in many phases, this act grows into a root of bitterness. What we fail to realize is that such animosity creates stress and anxiety that intensify whatever sickness we are dealing with. Not to minimize anyone's illness, but it has been proven that people tend to get better or worse depending on their attitude toward their condition. Joyful spirit people may carry an illness, but the illness hardly controls them. Those who know the power of their own tongue make proclamations that bring peace and hope. As human beings, we add so much more to the world than just a physical body, because we are spirit beings, created, called, and ordained with purposefulness to be used for the kingdom of God. Plans were set in place for our lives before we were ever birthed (Jeremiah 29:11). We have the capability to produce effective change in the hearts of others by our powerful words of encouragement. How often do we even consider the impact our relationship with others has on them as they deal with their seemingly impossible circumstances? My point is, all of us have something to give. I must admit hearing the scripture, "All things work together for the good of those who love God and are called to His purpose," doesn't set well when it looks as though hell is raging, but the moment we redirect our attention on helping others, murmuring will cease, pitting, or beating ourselves up will stop, a complete satisfaction arises, which puts us in the position to strength someone else.

It is imperative to be convinced of this one thing; pain cannot dictate the future. God has graced us to accomplish great things on the earth, "Greater works shall ye do..." he states in John 14:12. You can make a difference! Whether receiving or giving a vital organ to sustain life, it would be a sacrificial miracle. People are often curious about paraplegics as to what keeps them going in the absence of a limb or having uncountable surgeries to preserve life. Many would be eager to know what occurred, why and when. Like the man born blind in John 9:2, many people inquired, including Jesus' disciples, asking, "Who sinned?" Jesus answered the people, saying, "Neither this man nor his parents sinned, but this happened so that the works of God might be displayed in him." Have you ever considered yourself as one chosen to show forth the glory of God? You've seen individuals without a limb win marathons. They remained focused and determined to cross the finish line. Nick Vujicic is a TV evangelist who was born with tetra-amelia syndrome. He has no limbs, but he shares his story all over the world. He is a married man and a father.

It would have been a great thing if "in the beginning," God had made it possible enough for us to believe that He truly exists; however, it takes knowing and having a personal relationship. Acts and testimonies of God's faithfulness is the only confirmation we can own: that I once was blind, but now I see; lost but now found, to persuade people that God is truly real. Have you read about the four lepers? Leprosy, also known as Hansen's disease (HD), is a chronic infection caused by the bacteria Mycobacterium leprae and Mycobacterium lepromatous. In II Kings chapter seven, four lepers came to a decision within themselves while waiting on death and said: "Why sit here and die?" So, what can we do with the life we have? Yes, I'm sick, sick and tired of my pains; my hair is falling out, I am fed up with meds, but I am not alone. "If I can but touch the hem of Jesus' garment, I will be made whole." The Bible is full of awesome stories of God's miraculous interventions.

Another leper in Matthew 8:2 shows immediate restoration. It reads, "And a leper came to Him (Jesus) and bowed down before Him, and said, Lord, if You are willing, You can make me clean." Then Jesus stretched out His hand and touched the leper and said, "I am willing; be cleansed," immediately the leprosy was gone. Some were even healed as they went along (Luke 17:14). Imagine it is your worst day and all of a sudden you feel better, you're not sure when or what time the healing took place, meds didn't' do it nor doctors, all you know is, "I was sick and now I'm well." You name it HIV, Cancer, Lupus, Endometriosis, etc. Whatever it is, God is able to deliver us. It is not just what I read in the Bible, it is the Bible coming to life in me, the work of the Holy Spirit daily.

Possibly you have heard the saying, "Mind over matter." Well, having the mind of Christ and completely depending on Him means putting aside everything else we think matters. Whether you were born with or you are dealing with a condition or not (Philippians 2:5) let your mind be in agreement with Christ. The Bible declares all things are possible to him that believes. Nothing is impossible with God! Why not believe change is inevitable for you and others? God is amazing in how He upholds us in ways beyond our imagination. That alone brings testament to His awesome power. Taking a stand through faith even in frailness gives hope and boosts one's spirit of determination. What is unfortunate is to be born with critical illness before you've begun to live. How difficult it is to lie down well and wake up totally exasperated by some physical or mental disorder, and especially when life does not prepare you for the lump, the clot, the memory loss, or to birth a child with physical defects. These are real issues; nothing is being dismissed or minimized, doctors and hospitals around the world have given detailed reports that the power of prayer is a key component to physical and mental healing. As a volunteer chaplain for numerous years in a local hospital, when it comes to pain and suffering, all genders, ages, and races are included. Be it Black or White Americans, Hispanics, Muslims, Jews, and Gentiles, it does not matter, we are not exempt. Walking in love matters, and praying to God who so loves the world is the only answer.

In the pages ahead, you will read about a few illnesses that have been highlighted with personal testimonies from women who want you to know that you can overcome, live through, and survive. As you connect with the words, stories, and journeys of the women in this book, consider your grandmother, mom, sister, aunt, wife, daughter, or friend who needs to be uplifted, and encouraged to hope in not just a God, but Abba/Father. The God of grace, and mercy, His son Jesus who like you and many others suffered and died but resurrected to bring hope and a comforter, the Holy Spirit. Although I am not in your shoes nor you mine, let it be known we all have a story to tell of experiences we dread due to health and emotional issues. I enjoin us therefore to support one another in ways that give strength, encouragement, sisterhood, etc. by doing whatever it takes to make sure no one is left untouched while facing their struggle. If walking together is the answer, let's lock arms and keep moving one step at a time in the matchless compassion of a great God. And remember to watch your words, what you say, declare, and decree over your life means everything.

What you say can preserve life or destroy it; so you must accept the consequences of your words. Proverbs 18:21

October 13, 1979, an 8lb baby girl was birthed, my second child. She was absolutely beautiful. The doctor signed her off as healthy and strong to be three weeks short of nine months. Within six to eight weeks of life, her eyes could no longer focus on anything, they seemed to just stare without movement. Something was not right. You ever felt entirely helpless while searching for answers? After several tests, the diagnosis was in Hydrocephalus, which is a condition in which there is an abnormal buildup of CSF (cerebrospinal fluid) in the cavities (ventricles) of the brain. The buildup is often caused by an obstruction which prevents proper fluid drainage. The fluid buildup can raise intracranial pressure inside the skull which compresses surrounding brain tissues, possibly causing progressive enlargement of the head, convulsions, and brain damage. Hydrocephalus can be fatal if left untreated. Wow! Quite a bit to digest. Perfectly normal gorgeous baby-girl, yet within a few weeks of existence in this world, she lacked development in her brain. Sound the alarm! Nothing prepared us for the months ahead; we were just totally ignorant of the level of care it would take, or the many tests and hospital visits she would undergo. Someone dared to say she was brainless, but after testing and observation by one pediatrician, the report came back that her brain was tremendously damaged and from that point, the thought of her abnormality became a reality. Talking about confused and disturbed, the entire situation stimulated anger. As a Christian, I expected God at any time to jump right in, but to my bewilderment, He didn't, and my immaturity caused me to speak negative words. No answer to the whys in my heart. I blamed myself for doing something wrong or different than the last pregnancy. I blamed God for not showing up when I knew He could make her better. Jessica was her name, (one whom God beholds, one that lights up a room), her prognosis was not good, but her response to me proved to be hopeful. That was how our journey began. Jessica was later diagnosed with Cerebral Palsy, and this neurological disorder of the brain affected every area of Jessica's body. The fluid-filled her head to the size of a bed pillow; she never experienced the wonderful stages of rolling over, sitting up, crawling, and of course, those first baby steps that gave me joy while watching my other children and later witnessing my grandbabies, Kaylee, Samuel, and soon to be MacKenzie. It was very difficult from day to day putting in feeding tubes, observing seizures and the desire for her to live a normal life.

I longed to hear her say momma, but she could not. The good news was that she did have electric smiles that could fill anyone's heart. Jessica outlived the prognosis of being a vegetable as spoken over her life. As a matter of fact, she lived to be seven (7) years old. She attended school for special education, and her life produced some of my most treasured memories. The care it took to maintain Jessica's health drew me from my own personal issues and challenged me to see myself and my areas of weakness. So, instead of operating motherhood in self-pity, I put on my big girl panties, and moved forward while dealing with my marital problems. Not everyone even your close partner can cope with life-changing medical conditions. Thus, I grabbed the horn of single parenthood and made a decision to persevere.

Heartbreak turned triumph and the lessons, and experiences I gained can never be valued more highly. Jessica was a joyful test of strength. God took her back home, but she was His to take, and He left me with a remarkable memory of one of His fruits of the Spirit called long-suffering along with three other wonderful children to mother. Had I stayed sad, angry, and bitter and confused, I would have missed the blessing Jessica impressed upon my heart and probably neglect my other children, too. The journey my little girl and I shared together healed a deep emotional crevice in my heart and also gave me unspeakable joy I never knew of.

This title, God's Elect Ladies, calls women everywhere to rise up, communicate and make their stories known. God placed elect ladies in my heart years ago when I taught a Sunday school class of aggressive, beautiful, young female teens, youthful women filled with dreams and a desire to please God. Our objective was to have faith in whatever visions or goals sought out to achieve. Our motivation was "If I can help somebody as I travel along, cheer them with a word or song, then my living shall not be in vain," written in 1945 by Alma Bazel Androzzo, and made famous by Mahalia Jackson, a hit in 1951 for an Irish tenor, Joseph Locke. Some of the students have moved forward in spite of death wrenching physical conditions, and they are determined not to be stopped, for destiny in its completion still awaits them. "God's Elect Ladies" is a reminder that we are his chosen regardless of what we face in life, that we are called and equipped to stand, sometimes with a prop, but altogether well-built to survive whatever life throws at us. We are not ashamed to profess the love and power of God's grace as women; we are described as the "weaker vessel" in scripture though not in any way to demean nor insult us but a reality of our capacity to conceive, carry and birth out of the tenderness of our wombs. It does not mean weak-mindedness nor should we have to compete to prove just how strong we are. As elect women, the secret is to be whole. We are known by our inner strength and gentle spirit, we are thinkers, delivered from what has hindered us from fulfilling and carrying out God's will and assignment. And our assurance is that God is forever with us. We are his trophies to admire; our strategy is planning, pacing and positioning ourselves to move in the steps ordered by the Lord.

Whether your days are good or not so good, God is faithful; He just wants a surrendered heart, a heart He can be glorified through in sickness or in health, in riches or in poverty till death do us part. You may have been diagnosed of a particular illness but let not fear overwhelm you; educate yourself, take control, there are healthy choices you can make every day, such as choosing the right foods and friends. A healthful diet goes a long way, mixed with exercise, reading, being in positive environments, and understanding the people you hang around, talk to and mingle with also play an important role in affecting how we think and cope in everyday living. Know who you are and be that woman!

Listed are some diseases/illnesses I have become aware of from women in my circle:

Dementia – Dementia is not a specific disease. It is a descriptive term for a collection of symptoms that can be caused by a number of disorders that affect the brain. People with dementia have significantly impaired intellectual functioning that interferes with normal activities and relationships. They also lose their ability to solve problems and maintain emotional control, and they may experience personality changes and behavioral problems, such as agitation, delusions, and hallucinations. While memory loss is a common symptom of dementia, memory loss by itself does not mean that a person has dementia. Doctors diagnose dementia only if two or more brain functions – such as memory and language skills – are significantly impaired without loss of consciousness. Some of the diseases that can cause symptoms of dementia are Alzheimer's disease, vascular dementia, Lewy body dementia, frontotemporal dementia, Huntington's disease, and Creutzfeldt-Jakob disease. Doctors have identified other conditions that can cause dementia or dementia-like symptoms including reactions to medications, metabolic problems and endocrine abnormalities, nutritional deficiencies, infections, poisoning, brain tumors, anoxia or hypoxia (conditions in which the brain's oxygen supply is either reduced or cut off entirely), and heart and lung problems. Although it is common amongst very elderly individuals, dementia is not a normal part of aging process.

Aplastic anemia – Aplastic anemia is a condition that occurs when your body stops producing enough new blood cells. Aplastic anemia leaves you feeling fatigued and with a higher risk of infections and uncontrolled bleeding. A rare and serious condition, aplastic anemia, can develop at any age. Aplastic anemia may occur suddenly, or it can occur slowly and get worse over a long period of time. Treatment for aplastic anemia may include medications, blood transfusions or a stem cell transplant also known as a bone marrow transplant.

Endometriosis - Endometriosis is a female health disorder that occurs when cells from the lining of the womb (uterus) grow in other areas of the body. This can lead to pain, irregular bleeding, and problems getting pregnant (infertility). Endometriosis is a painful, chronic disease that affects at least 6.3 million women and girls in the U.S., 1 million in Canada, and millions more worldwide. It occurs when a tissue like that which lines the uterus (tissue called the endometrium) is found outside the uterus – usually in the abdomen, on the ovaries, fallopian tubes, and ligaments that support the uterus; the area between the vagina and rectum; the outer surface of the uterus; and the lining of the pelvic cavity. Other sites for these endometrial growths may include the bladder, bowel, vagina, cervix, vulva, and in abdominal surgical scars. Less commonly, they are found in the lung, arm, thigh, and other locations.

This misplaced tissue develops into growths or lesions that respond to the menstrual cycle in the same way that the tissue of the uterine lining does: each month the tissue builds up, breaks down, and sheds. Menstrual blood flows from the uterus and out of the body through the vagina, but the blood and tissue shed from endometrial growths have no way of leaving the body. This results in internal bleeding, a breakdown of the blood and tissue from the lesions, and inflammation – and can cause pain, infertility, scar tissue formation, adhesions, and bowel problems.

Alopecia - Alopecia areata is a type of hair loss that occurs when your immune system mistakenly attacks hair follicles. Alopecia (al-oh-PEE-shah) means hair loss. When a person has a medical condition called alopecia areata (ar-ee-AH-tah), their hair falls out in round patches. The hair can fall out on the scalp and elsewhere on the body. Alopecia areata can cause different types of hair loss. Each of these types has a different name:

- Alopecia areata (hair loss in patches).

- Alopecia-totalis (loss of all hair on the scalp).

- Alopecia universalis (loss of all hair on the body).

Hair often grows back but may fall out again. Sometimes the hair loss lasts for many years. Alopecia is not contagious. It is not due to nerves. What happens is that the immune system attacks the hair follicles (structures that contain the roots of the hair), causing hair loss.

Lupus - a chronic, inflammatory, autoimmune disease that can damage any part of the body (skin, joints, and/or organs inside the body). Lupus (also called systemic lupus erythematosus) is a disorder of the immune system. Normally, the immune system protects the body against invading infections and cancers. In lupus, the immune system is over-active and produces increased amounts of abnormal antibodies that attack the body's tissues and organs. Lupus can affect many parts of the body, including the joints, skin, kidneys, lungs, heart, nervous system, and blood vessels. The signs and symptoms of lupus differ from person to person; the disease can range from mild to life-threatening. Initial symptoms of lupus may begin with a fever, vascular headaches, epilepsy, or psychoses. A striking feature of lupus is a butterfly-shaped rash over the cheeks. In addition to a headache, lupus can cause other neurological disorders, such as mild cognitive dysfunction, organic brain syndrome, peripheral neuropathies, sensory neuropathy, psychological problems (including personality changes, paranoia, mania, and schizophrenia), seizures, transverse myelitis, and paralysis and stroke.

There is no cure for lupus. Treatment is symptomatic. With a combination of medication, rest, exercise, proper nutrition, and stress management, most individuals with lupus can often achieve remission or reduce their symptom levels. Medications used in the treatment of lupus may include aspirin and other nonsteroidal anti-inflammatory medications, antimalarials, corticosteroids, and immunosuppressive drugs.

Sickle Cell Anemia is a disease passed down through families. The red blood cells that are normally shaped like a disc take on a sickle or crescent shape. Red blood cells carry oxygen to the body.

Asthma is a disorder that causes the airways of the lungs to swell and narrow, leading to wheezing, shortness of breath, chest tightness, and coughing.

Multiple sclerosis is an unpredictable disease of the central nervous system. Multiple sclerosis (MS) can range from relatively benign to somewhat disabling to devastating, as communication between the brain and other parts of the body is disrupted. Many researchers believe MS to be an autoimmune disease – one in which the body, through its immune system, launches a defensive attack against its own tissues. In the case of MS, it is the nerve-insulating myelin that comes under assault. Such assaults may be linked to an unknown environmental trigger, perhaps a virus. Most people experience their first symptoms of MS between the ages of 20 and 40; the initial symptom of MS is often blurred or double vision, red-green color distortion, or even blindness in one eye. Most MS patients experience muscle weakness in their extremities and difficulty with coordination and balance. These symptoms may be severe enough to impair walking or even standing. In the worst cases, MS can produce partial or complete paralysis. Most people with MS also exhibit paresthesia, transitory abnormal sensory feelings such as numbness, prickling, or "pins and needles" sensations. Some may also experience pain. Speech impediments, tremors, and dizziness are other frequent complaints. Occasionally, people with MS have hearing loss. Approximately half of all people with MS experience cognitive impairments such as difficulties with concentration, attention, memory, and poor judgment, but such symptoms are usually mild and are frequently overlooked. Depression is another common feature of MS.

Cancer is the uncontrolled growth of abnormal cells in the body. Cancerous cells are also called malignant cells. Cancer develops when the body's normal control mechanism stops working. Old cells do not die, and cells grow out of control, forming new abnormal cells. Cancer can occur anywhere in the body. In women, breast cancer is most common. In men, it's prostate cancer. However, lung cancer and colorectal cancer affect both men and women in high numbers.

There are five main categories of cancer:

- ♣ Carcinomas begin in the skin or tissues that line the internal organs.

- ♣ Sarcomas develop in the bone, cartilage, fat, muscle or other connective tissues.

- ♣ Leukemia begins in the blood and bone marrow.

- ♣ Lymphomas start in the immune system.

Central nervous system cancers develop in the brain and spinal cord. Treatment options depend on the type of cancer, its stage, whether it has spread over the patient's body, and their general health. The goal of treatment is to kill as many cancerous cells while minimizing damage to normal cells nearby. Advances in technology make this possible.

The three main treatments are:

- ♣ Surgery: directly removing the tumor

- ♣ Chemotherapy: using chemicals to kill cancerous cells

♣ Radiation therapy: using X-rays to kill cancerous cells

The same cancer type in one individual can be very different from that cancer in another individual. Within a single type of cancer, such as breast cancer, researchers are discovering subtypes that each requires a different treatment approach.

What can you do to manage the side effects of cancer treatment?

Integrative oncology services describe a broad range of complementary treatments that combat side effects, boost the immune system and maintain well-being. Treating cancer cannot focus on the disease alone but must address the pain, fatigue, and depression that come with it.

Integrative oncology services include:

♣ Nutrition therapy to help prevent malnutrition and reduce side effects

♣ Naturopathic medicine to safely strengthen your immune system, boost your energy and reduce side effects

♣ Oncology rehabilitation to rebuild strength and overcome some of the physical effects of treatment

♣ Mind-body medicine to improve emotional well-being through counseling, stress management techniques, and support groups

What does the future hold for cancer treatment?

The future of cancer treatment lies in providing patients with an even greater level of personalization. Doctors are beginning to offer treatment options based on the genetic changes occurring in a specific tumor. An innovative new diagnostic tool, the genomic tumor assessment, examines a patient's tumor genetically to identify the mechanism that caused cancer. Genomic tumor assessment can result in a more personalized approach to cancer treatment.

Leukemia is cancer of the body's blood-forming tissues, including the bone marrow and the lymphatic system. Many types of leukemia exist. Some forms of leukemia are more common in children while its other forms occur mostly in adults. Leukemia usually involves the white blood cells. Your white blood cells are potent infection fighters — they normally grow and divide in an orderly way, as your body needs them. But in people with leukemia, the bone marrow produces abnormal white blood cells, which don't function properly. Treatment for leukemia can be complex — depending on the type of leukemia and other factors. But there are strategies and resources that can help to make your treatment successful.

Crohn Disease is named after Dr. Burrill B. Crohn, who first described the disease in 1932 along with colleagues, Dr. Leon Ginzburg, and Dr. Gordon D. Oppenheimer. Crohn's disease belongs to a group of conditions known as Inflammatory Bowel Diseases (IBD). Crohn's disease is a chronic inflammatory condition of the gastrointestinal tract. When reading about inflammatory bowel diseases, it is important to know that Crohn's disease is not the same thing as ulcerative colitis, another type of IBD. The symptoms of these two illnesses are quite similar, but the areas affected in the gastrointestinal tract (GI tract) are different. Crohn's most commonly affects the end of the small bowel (the ileum) and the beginning of the colon, but it may affect any part of the gastrointestinal (GI) tract, from the mouth to the anus. Ulcerative colitis is limited to the colon, also called the large intestine. Crohn's disease can also affect the entire thickness of the bowel wall, while ulcerative colitis only involves the innermost lining of the colon. Finally, in Crohn's disease, the inflammation of the intestine can "skip"-- leaving normal areas in between patches of diseased intestines. In ulcerative colitis, this does not occur. Crohn's disease can affect any part of the GI tract.

Cerebral Palsy refers to any one of a number of neurological disorders that appear in infancy or early childhood and permanently affect body movement and muscle coordination but don't worsen over time. Even though cerebral palsy affects muscle movement, it isn't caused by problems in the muscles or nerves. It is caused by abnormalities in parts of the brain that control muscle movements. The majority of children with cerebral palsy are born with it, although it may not be detected until months or years later. The early signs of cerebral palsy usually appear before a child reaches 3 years of age. And the most common of its signs are a lack of muscle coordination when performing voluntary movements (ataxia); stiff or tight muscles and exaggerated reflexes (spasticity); walking with one foot or leg dragging; walking on the toes, a crouched gait, or a "scissor" gait; and muscle tone that is either too stiff or too floppy. A small number of children have cerebral palsy as the result of brain damage in the first few months or years of life, brain infections such as bacterial meningitis or viral encephalitis, or head injury from a motor vehicle accident, a fall, or child abuse.

Cerebral palsy can't be cured, but treatment will often improve a child's capabilities. In general, the earlier treatment begins, the better chance children have of overcoming developmental disabilities or learning new ways to accomplish the tasks that challenge them. Treatment may include physical and occupational therapy, speech therapy, drugs to control seizures, relax muscle spasms, and alleviate pain; surgery to correct anatomical abnormalities or release tight muscles; braces and other orthotic devices; wheelchairs and rolling walkers; and communication aids such as computers with attached voice synthesizers.

Researchers are investigating the roles of mishaps early in brain development, including genetic defects, which are sometimes responsible for the brain malformations and abnormalities that result in cerebral palsy. Scientists are also looking at traumatic events in newborn babies' brains, such as bleeding, epileptic seizures, and breathing and circulation problems, which can cause the abnormal release of chemicals that trigger the kind of damage that causes cerebral palsy. Researchers also hope to find ways to prevent white matter disease--the most common cause of cerebral palsy. To make sure children are getting the right kinds of therapies, studies are also being done that evaluate both experimental treatments and treatments already in use so that physicians and parents have valid information to help them choose the best therapy.

National Institute of Neurological Disorders and Stroke

National Institutes of Health

Bethesda, MD 20892

http:// ninds.nih.gov

American Cancer Society

National Home Office

250 Williams Street, NW

Atlanta, GA 30303-1002

Tel: 800-ACS-2345 (227-2345)

http://www.cancer.org

Cancer Care

275 Seventh Avenue

New York, NY 10001

Tel: Business: 212-712-8400 Services: 800-813-HOPE (4673)

Fax: 212-712-8495

Email: info@cancercare.org http://www.cancercare.org

Cancer Treatment Centers of America Global, Inc.

General Inquiries: 561-923-3100

Media Inquiries: 561-923-3198

Sponsorship Requests and Contributions: 561-923-3149

Crohn's & Colitis Foundation of America (CCFA)

http://www.ccfa.org/what-are-crohns-and-colitis/

Endometriosis Association International Headquarters

8585 North 76th Place

Milwaukee, WI 53223 USA

http://www.endometriosisassn.org/

Mayo Clinic

13400 E. Shea Blvd.

Scottsdale, AZ 8525

CHAPTER ONE

Momma-Mary

Dementia, our family have seen firsthand the loss of brain function that occurs with this disease. It affects memory, thinking, language, judgment, and behavior. In my research of dementia, the word gets used quite a bit when discussing aging and certain diseases like Alzheimer's. What is true about dementia? The facts are, it carries a set of symptoms, a traumatic blow of the head, which I recall Mom speaking about when she experienced a car accident on the interstate years ago, as well as other causes of disorders. However, witnessing them firsthand can be disturbing and can give the feel of helplessness to your loved ones.

Momma Mary, a mother, sister, aunt, and grand/great-grandmother, lived with dementia, though her daily routine changed rather rapidly in the last few years of her life. After retirement, her days were not as busy as they had been, nonetheless, she always found places to go and to attend to people who needed her care. After a while, her life, as we knew it, began dwindling, her lack of memory in what seemed like simple everyday conversations became alarming, and the things she could not remember caused an emotional scare among her children, my siblings. We were not ready for this reality, but it did not alter the symptoms; life was changing, and we were being warned. Dementia began slowly, easing its way into her life, the transformation of behavior was unexplainable. The truth is, we didn't even know to call it dementia; however, the diagnosis was clear, and it was noted as a part of aging. Over time, things we took for granted like hygiene, making a cup of coffee, cooking, etc., which Mom did so well, steered us into looking at the situation more seriously and intentionally about how we ministered daily care because we were facing a new norm. Life not only appeared worse, but our anxiety about Mom's condition also unleashed great concern. The signs began to jump out at us here and there; frustration escalated as we shared in her deficiency to remember what day it was, whether or not she took her medication, or recalling some of the grandchildren by name, so much became troubling for her and us. To adjust and understand from both perspectives would be a great topic of discussion among so many families. The abnormality of watching your mom or any loved one transform before your eyes is and was a very painful experience to us. And expressing our feelings was even more perplexing; we lacked understanding, some in denial, or fretful, even fearful of what was happening.

Momma Mary could be pretty stubborn at times, having all those years of nursing under her belt, and she felt as if she knew what was best for her. Nevertheless, the more I think about her adjusting to her new realities, the more it occurs to me that it could have been very challenging to her. She loved her family, and her reactions to her new self was to not be a burden. However, we knew she could not make serious decisions alone. How hard it must have been recalling the memory of things such as what day it was or the many times she asked, "Where am I?" This change took place in a woman who was lively and sharp, a hard worker, and a woman who put others before herself. She was always extremely vibrant and full of life, even when we desired for her to slow down, or take it easy, she was always determined to get her jobs done or finish her tasks. Laziness was at no time a part of her character, and you were never on her watch. My siblings and cousins, I'm sure, would agree to these evergreen memories. Growing up, Mom had such an order about things; how we cleaned, cooked, what we wore and how we presented ourselves at home and in public. She was a devoted prayer-woman. Her caring attitude toward so many, young and old, is one of my greatest memories. Even when she fussed, there always remained love so deep in her, love to make sure none of her loved ones were left behind, but that all would strive for the highest achievements. As a nursing technician in the hospital for several years, she served the community and still found time to make sure we had a spiritual foundation to build our lives upon. She loved hard and sacrificed much to keep from revealing her own hurt most of the time, always wanting to do more. Unfortunately, many family members kept their distance as she embraced senior living, not understanding her necessity of the human touch, or the need to be needed for whatever she could give. Like most seniors, she loved and missed her grand and great-grandchildren. What a difference they can make in the lives of elderly persons and how they light up a room with such sincerity! The communication her family labeled as fussing seemed to delay or shorten visits, but truth be told, it was bitterness toward her own personal struggles and the heartaches life had dealt her that she found hard to face, not wanting any of her family to fall into the same pitfalls. Be that as it may, some might still say it pushed them away or caused them to avoid coming around altogether, but then again, maybe we didn't allow ourselves the opportunity to deeply know her beyond the surface, maybe we were more concerned with our own feelings. The stories Mom shared were not always favorable, as a matter of fact, they were painful sometimes and always left her in a place of ache, but her heart always reached out. She had a favorite word of counsel for the young and indeed all who came in contact with her; namely, "Romance without finance is ignorance." Obviously, she didn't want us to be caught up in stupidity, thinking we were in love with someone or an idea that would leave us in financial struggle. Of course, if we were poor growing up, we didn't know it because we always had a roof over our heads, and anyone who came to our house could always eat. In her later years, she sometimes felt abandoned, which ordinarily hurts at any stage of life. Why am I saying all of these? Well, some of you reading this story may come to face similar challenges with your loved ones, and Mom would want you to be prepared. She would want you to know that the strong is often misunderstood; you know, the one who seeks healing for everyone else but never takes enough time for themselves. On October 3rd, 2016, she turned 80 years old. I dare not say that loudly, but what a blessing! Truthfully speaking, sharing time together helps patients like Mom to regain memory, because they identify with whom they see, touch, and hear, which brings about a tremendous difference in day-to-day living. It allows them to reminiscence.

Momma Mary resided in a senior living health facility whereas she participated in daily therapy for walking and recreation. She really had more life within her than she wanted to admit. Interacting with her peers was also helpful. Even though her brain had been affected by these symptoms of dementia, the mother I know was a fighter. Momma Mary birthed seven children and raised ten plus. The traumatic car accident she experienced on the interstate years ago that left her lying on the side of the road for quite a while, as she usually told us, led to surgery and the correction of a disc in her neck. Maybe this was the cause of some of her discomforts, I don't know. It is noted that brain damage from an injury or a stroke can also influence dementia, as can other symptoms, we just don't have all the answers.

If Mom was writing this story, I believe she would say her biggest fear in the duration of this illness was loneliness; she never wanted to be left alone. But as she had taught us, we rehearsed the same words in her ears, "God will never leave us nor forsake us." "For God so loved the world that He gave His only begotten son…." This remains a message to us all, one we can rest upon. Mom was a blessed woman and a trailblazer. Whatever roads of trial we have faced or will face, she has gone through them before us, showing us that the strength we need to survive is in Christ Jesus our Lord. We salute you, Mom, for your love and faithfulness.

Aplastic anemia: Wow! Just when I thought this chapter was complete, Mom was taken to the hospital, and her blood count had dropped extremely low. Thus, a bone marrow biopsy was done, which involved the insertion of a needle directly into the pelvic bone to withdraw marrow for examination under the microscope. She was diagnosed of Aplastic anemia associated with bone cancer, a condition that occurs when your body stops producing enough new blood cells. *Aplastic anemia* leaves you feeling fatigued and with a higher risk of infections and uncontrolled bleeding. It is a rare and serious condition that can develop at any age. Our grandmother, and Mom's mother experienced Aplastic anemia also. I remember my sister and me helping Mom care for her years ago.

The family met again to deliberate, and this time, hospice was invited for support and comfort. Did Mom know she would reach this point in her health? We all wondered. Is this a heredity gene we should be concerned about? Mom returned to the health center, but after a while of being there, she revisited the hospital, and her emergency confirmed that the infection had spread throughout her entire body. After doctors reassured the family that all had been done, Mom returned to the health center to live out her days. Sadly enough, within a couple of months, her eyes closed to never open again. As she died, she muttered some unclear words. She lived the last days of her life at the health center. Mom is gone, but her life lives on in us. Early Friday morning while preparing to travel to Georgia, I stopped to visit Mom, but she was asleep, and I didn't want to wake her. I kissed her forehead before leaving and on May 20, 2017, I was sitting in my dad's living room in Georgia when the call came that Mom had slept away into eternity. She went home to be with the Lord. Oh, how grateful we are that God blessed her life and ours!

CHAPTER TWO

Yokasta

My **Alopecia** Story: It is often said, "Beauty is in the eye of the beholder." However, what if your appearance challenges every known standard of beauty that exists? What if your appearance changes drastically, with no warning whatsoever? Finally, what if your drastic change in appearance irrevocably changes the way you relate to friends, family, and the world around you?

This is the reality faced by the 140 million people around the world – 6.5 million people in the United States alone – living with alopecia areata (AA), an autoimmune skin and hair disorder that causes hair loss. The severity of hair loss in patients with alopecia ranges from patchy hair loss (alopecia areata) to total scalp hair loss (alopecia totalis) and all the way to complete body hair loss (alopecia universalis), including eyelashes and eyebrows. Alopecia areata is not contagious, nor is it life-threatening. However, for the millions of people around the world who suffer from this disease, the onset of alopecia is psychologically traumatic for the patient, in addition to their loved ones, who may never show symptoms of the disease themselves.

I was diagnosed with alopecia areata in 1984, two years after the appearance of the first bald spot in my head at age 4. The following account is my own story of alopecia, from the early days of the unknown to the present day, and the long journey to unconditional self-acceptance I took along the way.

My first clue that something was wrong came one winter morning, as I was getting ready for school. We were following our established routine, and I was having my pigtails fixed when suddenly my mother stopped what she was doing and took me into the bathroom and looked at my head under a brighter light. After a moment, she told me not to move and then went into my bedroom and proceeded to my bedroom, took the pillowcases off my pillows and removed the sheets and blankets from my bed, turned them inside out, and shook them thoroughly. She then ran out of the room and checked the bathroom and kitchen drawers. I watched all this with a growing sense of confusion and a growing feeling that something was not right. Finally, my mother came into the room where she left me with my grandmother and asked me if I had been pulling on my hair at all. I told her that I hadn't. She then asked me if I had been playing with any scissors or knives at all. Because I knew those items were not toys and I was not allowed to play with them. I answered no. (And I really hadn't been playing with them.) Finally, she asked me if I had been allowing my classmates to play with my hair. I told her that I hadn't.

While she was asking me these questions, my grandmother was looking at my head, examining my scalp to see if there were any cuts or bruises there to explain what I now know were the first alopecia areata spots in my head. My grandmother, who was a former nurse and a very practical person, got a seamstress' tape measure and measured the size of the two spots in my head. They measured the size of a dime and the size of a quarter. The smaller of the two spots was located at the top of my head, near my hairline, and the larger of the two was in the back of my head, close to the nape of my neck. Because my hair was very long and thick at the time, the spots were easily covered up. My grandmother advised my mother to watch my hair for a couple of weeks to see if the spots would grow back in by themselves. They never did. In fact, they got worse.

After approximately six weeks had passed, the two initial spots grew to the size of half-dollars, and more spots appeared as well. It was during this time that my mother started this weird kind of comb-over with a side ponytail in the top of my head to cover those spots and a smaller ponytail in the back to cover the spot at the nape of my neck. It was also during this time that we started the first of a long journey to numerous doctors, each of which asked my parents more questions than they provided answers to. I first went to see one Dr. Hamilton at Park View (now Centennial) Medical Center in Nashville, TN, who started me on a regimen of steroid creams that had to be rubbed in the morning and in the evening. I remember trying cream after cream and noticing my hair start growing again, only to fall out after about 2-3 months. Worse still, each time my hair started falling out again, I lost a little more hair.

The next doctor I visited was Dr. Johnson, at Meharry Medical College in Nashville, TN. It is important for me to note here that being a resident of Nashville at the time enabled my parents to seek the best medical care available, care which I might not have had had we remained in Norfolk, VA much longer. Nashville has long been viewed as a healthcare center in the South, and people come from all over the United States and all over the world to consult with the doctors at such noted institutions as Vanderbilt University, Meharry Medical College, and Centennial Medical Center. Dr. Johnson, although kind, was also unable to tell my parents definitively what the cause of my hair loss was, although he did remove me from the long regimen of steroids that Dr. Hamilton had prescribed – which had long since stopped working – and prescribed a topical ointment called Dritho-Scalp, which had a bit more success. By this time, I was 5 years old and completely bald.

I think it is a remarkable ability for a small child to focus only on the here and now, rather than the long-term effects a major life change can have. Initially, when the first spots started appearing in my head, I just accepted it, taking it as something that just happened, which Mommy and Daddy and Honey would take care of. And that was that. It did not exist for me anymore.

My mother, always overprotective in the best of circumstances, and my grandmother, to whom I was the center of the universe, immediately became more overprotective. Because both women were and still are very conscious of and obsessed with their image in the eyes of others, they forbade me to leave the house at any time without my head covered up, and any mention of my hair loss in public was prohibited. Because we were dealing with an unknown state of affairs in terms of what was causing my hair loss and what could be done about it, my mother and grandmother initially decided upon using scarves to cover up the baldness. They purchased several scarves in colors to match my school uniform and life continued. My classmates, all of whom lived in my neighborhood and went to my church, noticed the changes very gradually, for which I am very thankful. Because they saw the very gradual progression of my alopecia, from one spot to two and beyond, and because we were being educated in a loving, Christian environment that taught us to look past physical differences, I honestly cannot say that I recall being teased or picked on during those first years.

However, with the intuition only a child can have, I began to pick up the feeling that my baldness was something embarrassing to many people, and that made me feel ashamed to be the cause of the embarrassment. I think those early feelings of shame and embarrassment – the need to hide my problem – coupled with my own natural talents and the desire to show them off were the catalysts that fueled my desire to be known for something other than my hair loss. So I threw myself into my schoolwork. I finished my homework assignments faster and more often than my older classmates, with very few or no errors. When I was done, I always asked for more work. I asked to join my school's Academic Olympics team, which was made up primarily of 3rd, 4th, 5th, and 6th graders. I entered and won my school's oratory contest at age 6 with a speech of my own writing, becoming the youngest person in school history to do so. However, as the trophies and awards started to pile up and accumulate, so did the feeling that it still was not good enough, and it showed because my hair stubbornly refused to come back. Looking back on it now, I think it might have continued this way forever had it not been for a breakthrough and the intervention of some wonderful people.

The Breakthrough

In the summer of 1985, my parents were referred to Dr. Dana Latour, a very prominent dermatologist at Vanderbilt University Medical Center whose specialty was pediatric hair loss. My parents took me to the first appointment, and naturally, we were all apprehensive about what its outcome would be. I think that by this time we were all fearful that like the other doctors we had seen, Dr. Latour would not be able to come up with a diagnosis that could explain the baldness and that it would all just be a waste of time. However, we were in for a surprise. Dr. Latour came into the examining room, took one look at my head, looked at my fingernails, and said immediately to my parents, "Your child has alopecia areata." I remember the feeling of a huge weight being lifted from the room with those five words.

Finally, there was a diagnosis! This was what we had been searching two years for! Then the other shoe fell. My mother, being a woman of action, started asking the questions anyone would ask after receiving a diagnosis. "What is the cure? What are the treatments available? Is it contagious? Will the same thing happen to my other babies? Why does this happen?" Just one statement opened the floodgates of curiosity, and the questions swirled around waiting to be answered. Then Dr. Latour spoke.

She told my parents that there were very few effective treatments available and that there was no cure for alopecia. No, the condition is not contagious. It was impossible to tell if my sister would develop alopecia, and as far as why alopecia happens. Well, she couldn't answer that question any better than any other doctor, simply because they didn't know. After going over my medical history and asking questions about the Dritho-Scalp I had been using faithfully – which by then, to nobody's surprise, had stopped working – she took me off the ointment and actually prescribed sunlight and fun. She was the first person to suggest a wig for me to wear to school too.

She gave us the name of Dean's Wig Villa in Madison, TN, and its proprietress, Faye, with the recommendation to call her to set up an appointment to see her.

To my six-year-old eyes, Faye was an angel. She had this amazing waist-length silvery blond hair that hung loose and straight, and it was so thick! Her blue eyes were very understanding, and I remember her tearing up the very first time she looked at my bald head in her shop. She told my mother and my grandmother (my father had been sent back overseas by this time) that I was the youngest client she had ever had, but she promised my mother that she would do everything she could to help me find a hairstyle that everyone would like, but she was the first person to make it very clear that as much as everyone wanted to have an opinion about a wig, ultimately the final choice was MY decision and mine alone. I must have spent hours at a time over the next several weeks trying out different styles and lengths – it felt like I was playing dress up, but it was really real. Because children's wigs simply did not exist in 1985, there was an additional challenge: "How do you create a wig for a child, small enough to fit her head yet with enough room to grow as she grows?" Faye came up with a remarkable solution: She ordered adult-sized wigs and then cut them down herself to fix exactly to my head. This she did with the help of a plaster-cast mold of my head that she made so that she could work when I wasn't around. Then she took the excess hair that she had removed and then hand-tied it back into the smaller, YoKasta-sized wig to give it added fullness and styling versatility. This would allow me to wear pigtails, a ponytail, loose hair; you name it. Finally, the day arrived when my first new wig was ready. I wore it home and hung it on the wig head that Faye gave me for it, excited that I could go to school looking like everyone else the next day. It was like Christmas had come early – and I was eager to share my happiness with everyone. On top of that, my mother told my sisters and me that we were going to have another baby – maybe even a brother! I scarcely remember having a happier day than that one!

Differences can be devastating

The first day I wore my new wig to school, I was very excited. Now that I looked just like everyone else, I could go about the business of just being a kid, not "a kid with some issues." As I was heading for the chapel that first Monday morning, some of the students in the hallway stared, but I didn't realize it for what it was just yet. One or two students asked me if my hair had grown back over the holidays, and in my naïveté, I proudly told them that I had gotten a wig, so I could have hair just like them. I was answered with a strange look, and suddenly I began to feel that maybe – just maybe – telling everyone that I had new hair might not have been the best idea. That feeling was justified as my class entered the chapel and took our usual seats in front. As we passed everyone, I heard their whispers, and from the corner of my eye, I saw some students pointing and even heard a snicker or two.

Even though Caron, my best friend at the time, told me that everything was fine, I began to doubt her, especially when someone behind us said: "Look, it's a wig!" It was at that moment that I felt true embarrassment and shame – embarrassed because apparently my wig very obviously looked like a wig (to a child's eyes) and shame because I had to wear the wig in the first place. Even now, more than 20 years later, I cannot recall this event without tears coming to my eyes and having to pause for a moment because the shame and embarrassment was and is so overwhelming that my heart hurts to think about it. My reaction now is the same as my reaction then. I became very red-faced and hung my head, and quite sincerely wished that the floor would have opened up and swallowed me whole. I honestly don't recall the rest of the chapel service that first morning, but I do know that I would not have made it through that service without Caron holding my hand and reassuring me that everything would be fine.

When we returned to the classroom, my teacher made me come to the front of the classroom. When I got there, she gave a short lecture to the classroom about how differences made everyone unique and how special we all were. She admonished the class that just because I came to school looking different than I normally did; it did not mean that I was any different than I was before the holiday break. She also made it very clear that any teasing or bullying or excessive questions would not be tolerated in her classroom. Even though I was somewhat accustomed to being in the spotlight for my academic achievements, this was a spotlight I didn't want to be in. I would rather have just returned to the classroom and continued with my day as if nothing had happened. Instead, more attention was brought to my head than I was comfortable with, and I was certain that I wouldn't like what was going to happen after that.

The response of my classmates to the situation did not change overnight, but it did change. It started on the playground. Normally, when playing a team sport, I would be one of the first people chosen to a team. After I started wearing my wig, I very quickly became one of the last chosen. The girls in my classroom would make up clubs to be in, and when I asked if I could join, I would be told that I wasn't invited or that they had enough people and I would make it too many. The boys, never ones to willingly play with girls at that age anyway, would just pretend that I didn't exist. Pretty soon, it deteriorated into an alopecic child's worst nightmare: I was allowed to join in the team games and sports but at the cost of my wig being pulled off and covered up with the excuse of "it was an accident." Because I was always a bookish sort, telling my parents that I was being mistreated on the playground didn't help. Their response was to remind me that kids will be kids on the playground and that I needed to socialize. If I socialized, then eventually everyone would accept me for who I was. Eventually, I came to dread recess and physical education classes, so much so that I would pretend to be sick just so I could go to the library and be left in peace to read to my heart's content.

I found my refuge during those first years in the library. In the library, I could sit in peace and quiet and read wonderful books and magazines about past and present situations. I could transport myself into worlds where my wig and my alopecia didn't exist. In the stories I read, I was just me. I was accepted. I was everyone's friend. I think the librarian understood why I was there every day, and because she was sympathetic, she started pointing me toward the sections of the library that I hadn't yet explored. My librarian introduced me to Ovid, Homer, Plato, and Shakespeare. Bullfinch's Mythology became a constant companion and eventually, I was able to engage in conversations about writing techniques and different uses of imagery, satire, and allegory to illustrate certain points or shed light on a particular situation. While I hated and feared the very thought of going to recess, I looked forward to the time in the library and wished that I could always go to the library. When I went back to class after the recess hour, my classmates would not only start to crack jokes about my bald head and having to cover it up, but they would also tease me even more because they thought I was being kept inside because I was being punished. Ironically, I could withstand the teasing for being kept indoors a lot better than I could withstand being teased about my hair because only I knew the real reason I stayed inside. This might have continued the rest of the time that I was in school. I had a double blow of my sister starting kindergarten and my mother's surprise visit to the school changed everything again.

My mother, who had become suspicious of my sudden continuous return from school as neat and clean as I had been each morning I left home, decided one day to pay a surprise visit to the school to see just what I was doing at recess every day. She arrived unannounced and asked the recess teacher where I could be found. The recess teacher, who presumed that my mother already knew where I was, answered, "She's in the library – where she always is at this time." My mother then proceeded to come and collect me from the library and deposit me on the playground. As an added punishment, she took my books away and told me I couldn't have them back until after recess. That day I threw my first temper tantrum. I kicked and screamed and told her that I was not going to play with anyone who picked at me and teased me and pulled my wig off. Because the other children automatically pleaded their innocence, and because nobody else would come forward as an eyewitness, my protests were merely ignored. My response to that was to just simply come outside and sit on the fence at the farthest edge of the playground. If I could become invisible to my classmates, then maybe I could escape the hell of going to recess. For the most part, it worked. I became invisible to everyone for the hour we had to spend outside, but the teasing resumed as soon as we came inside.

When we were at home, my sister was my closest friend. My sister and I, from then until now, are complete opposites in everything from looks to personalities. Whereas I am fair-skinned with light eyes and blonde (except for my sudden baldness), she has dark hair, dark eyes, and olive skin. In fact, when we were younger, most people mistook her for being Indian or some other type of exotic child. Our personalities are just as different as our looks. Whereas I am normally very bubbly and outgoing, she is more reserved and quieter. You could read every emotion on my face and in my voice, but on hers, you usually see nothing and hear only a monotone. Where I generally tend to avoid conflict, she leaps into the fracas feet first. However, this is only a disguise for her. Despite her calm exterior, my sister is very observant, and in school, she noticed how upset I had become over going to school every day. Seeing how losing my hair had completely changed who I was and made me a withdrawn shell of who I had been before, she became fiercely protective of me. So, when she started school at the same school and saw for herself how I was being mistreated by the other children, fireworks were inevitable.

Either it could be considered ironic or a case of divine intervention depending on how you see it. By this, I mean the occurrence that my sister's recess time happened to be at the same time as my mine. This meant that our two classes shared the playground at the same time, which allowed my sister to see with her own eyes what was going on. For my part, I was truly happy again, because I knew that if nobody else would play with me, my sister would, and she always did. As far as she was concerned – well, remember the phrase, "Hell hath no fury like a woman scorned"? Well, modify that phrase to "hell hath no fury like my sister witnessing her sister being picked on" and you get a general picture of her reaction. Pretty soon, my parents and my grandmother started getting calls from the school on a daily basis about my sister. My parents were at a loss. She was such a sweet, quiet child at home. She never caused problems. Maybe she was having problems adjusting to school. Or just maybe the teachers were exaggerating about what was going on. Once again, my mother took it upon herself to pay an unannounced visit to the school to see what was going on for herself.

Nothing could have prepared my mother for what she saw that day. With her own eyes, she saw my classmates teasing me, picking on me, and on this particular day, a group of girls had pulled off my wig and was tossing it amongst themselves. Suddenly, there was a flash of black and green, and there was my sister, fighting each one of them like a lioness protecting her cub. The ferocity that she displayed – the righteous fury she felt – only that could have enabled her to rush headlong into that group of girls and attack them in the manner that she did. The other children on the playground could only stand there in stunned silence, too startled by the suddenness of the event to really respond. The only thing that could be heard on that playground was a couple of whimpers and moans and an enraged kindergartener yelling, "STAY AWAY FROM MY SISTER!!" That yell spurred my mother and the teachers into action. Somehow, they managed to extract both my sister and me from the melee and get us separated from the rest of the children. Once we got back inside the building and into the principal's office, my mother immediately rounded on the principal and demanded to know why the other children were being allowed to pick on me. However, before the principal could respond, I spoke up and stopped everyone dead in their tracks.

"Momma, I tried to tell you they were picking on me, but you didn't listen. You made me go to recess anyway. You let them pick on me." Dr. Graves, the principal, asked me what I thought would be the best thing to do to get everyone to stop teasing me. Even then I knew that the teasing, taunting, and bullying would never stop, and to presume that would be foolish in the extreme. However, because both my sister and I were smaller than the other children in my class (remember that I was two years – in some cases, three – years younger than the rest of my class) continuing to fight them was going to be an exercise in futility. So I took the only sure-fire escape route I had: I told the principal that I wanted to go back to the library.

The principal, ever the negotiator, asked my sister if that would make her stop fighting my classmates. My sister, seeing the question for the trap it was, answered, "Only if the other kids stop picking on my sister. If they pick on my sister, then I'm going to make them stop because YOU won't." Seeing that the conversation was going nowhere with my sister, the principal asked my mother to take us both home for the rest of the day, if for no other reason than to give everyone a timeout. Because it was a Friday, that meant she and I could start our weekend early. My mother agreed to this but also made it very clear that she expected the recess/playground issue to be resolved by the time we returned on Monday. It wasn't of course, and the issue was never resolved until we left that school for good. What did come of the incident, however, was that my mother's eyes were finally opened to the fact that in school, it's never a good thing to be different – especially for me.

What are you thinking, my dear?

Obviously, the school was more difficult than my parents had imagined. Unfortunately, I couldn't stop that unhappiness from carrying over into my home life as well. I stopped going outside with my sisters and chose to keep myself in my room with my books. I stopped asking to go places with my grand-mother, my aunts, and uncles, even my parents. If my parents wanted to go somewhere, the first question I asked was if I had to wear my wig or cover my head. If the answer was yes, then I didn't want to go. This meant that I hardly went anywhere unless I had to because my mother's answer to that question was ALWAYS yes. When my brother was born, my joy at having a baby brother was tempered by the fear that I had to go out in public and expose my head. My way around that was to convince my grandmother to take my sisters and me to the hospital at night before visiting hours ended, so I saw as few people as possible. My sisters started to complain that I never wanted to play with them or anyone else, and after a while, the neighbors presumed that my parents had only three children instead of 4, because I simply disappeared. At school, however, I was totally different. My classmates teased me, picked on me, and generally bullied me to no end; however, I basked in the glow of academic achievement. I lived my life for each and every academic contest that I entered; whether it be essay writing, speech giving, general quiz, bowl knowledge, you name it – I found a way to enter the contest and not only win but completely destroy my competitors.

During these very difficult years, one person remained my constant friend and companion and taught me more about acceptance and self-worth than anyone I ever knew. That person was my father, Michael. My father was a bookish sort, like me. Raised in California's foster care system off and on throughout his childhood and separated from his sisters for much of that time, he understood my feelings of loneliness and isolation during those years. My father, always a gentle-hearted, generous man, and with the protectiveness of any father, absorbed my pain as his own and often went out of his way to make sure that he didn't treat me any differently than anyone else. His approach to this was a study of contrasts. Where my mother and grandmother always insisted on my keeping my head covered when going out in public, my father would ask me what I wanted to wear. If I said that I wanted to go bare-headed, then he would accept that decision without question, and we would go on our way. If someone chose to stare a little too long, he would ask them if they wanted to ask me something and wait for an answer. This prompted me to tell the gawker about alopecia, what it did, and that of course, it was impolite to stare for too long without getting the facts. When we went on school field trips, my father was always the classroom parent, going just as much to experience the joy of field trips he never got to take in his own childhood as he was to keep me company. The most memorable field trip I ever took with my father was to the Masterworks art exhibit at the Tennessee State Museum in 1990. This collection, from the Bridgestone Museum of Art in Tokyo, Japan, houses hundreds of priceless works of art by Monet, Manet, Pissarro, Renoir, Degas, Picasso, Rembrandt, Raphael, Van Gogh, Reubens, and others considered being the most remarkable artists in history. We spent hours perusing each and every one of the paintings, discussing what we liked the most about the paintings. That one day I spent with my father I will always cherish, for it seemed like a culmination of the lessons he taught me about decision-making, self-reliance, and respect for others. My father was the one who laid the foundation for what to look for in a romantic relationship. He was the one who gave me the traditional "birds and the bees" talk and was the first person to present the possible reality that AA could possibly be something I would live with for the rest of my life. Although he also didn't focus on this, he wanted me to be prepared on how to deal with my AA when I hit puberty and all its changes.

In school, we learn about the opposite sex when puberty hits. We form our first romantic relationships, and the joy of having a first love is one of the rites of passage for any teen. I never had any interest in boys in school. For one thing, I had nothing in common with anyone I went to school with, let alone the boys, who sometimes teased me worse than the girls did. For another, it was always drilled into my ears by my parents and my grandmother that there was plenty of time to be interested in boys; my focus in school should be on school and nothing else. Plus, I never felt I was pretty enough to be seen by any boys as pretty, or even dateable. This has followed me into adulthood, and I still struggle with this belief daily.

…It grew back!

In the summer of 1991, as I was about to enter the 9th grade, I found myself in an interesting situation – literally overnight, my hair had grown back!!! I now found myself in the position of figuring out how to fix my own hair on a daily basis – learning how to use a curling iron, rollers, how to part my own hair straight, what type of brushes worked best on my hair type (it was very curly), and color or not to color.

It was very interesting to enter high school with a head full of long, dark hair. (After all those years of drugs and treatments, my hair was almost black instead of the blonde-haired girl my before-alopecia pictures showed.) Most of the students that I had gone to school with actually did not recognize me with hair, and their first and unanimous question was, "Is that hair yours?" Actually, truth be told, high school with hair – to me, anyway – was a lot less traumatic than it was for a lot of people. Once my hair grew back, the worst I had to worry about in school was whether or not someone was trying to be my friend to get the homework answers or because they thought I was cool.

I will not say I was the most popular person in school during those years because I definitely was not. However, once I stopped caring about whether or not I fit in with everyone, I did notice a substantial increase in my popularity amongst my peers. Was it because I wasn't trying so hard to be liked? Was it because of my hair? During my junior and the first half of my senior year, I relaxed enough to not let my hair be the driving force in my life. I colored my hair for the first time, and I almost believed that my hair would never fall out again.

It is a dangerous thing to grow up with less-than-realistic expectations, and it can be devastating when the reality of your expectations is significantly less than what you planned. I found this lesson out in the spring of 1995 when I discovered that dreaded spot. A single spot that caused the world to fall out from under my feet. Surprisingly enough, I wasn't scared or nervous, or even alarmed that my hair was falling out again. What was bothersome, though, was the speed with which my hair fell out this time. When my hair initially fell out at age 4, it took nearly a year for it to be totally gone.

This time, it was gone completely by June. In May, when I graduated from high school, I had blended what was left of my hair into a wig to disguise my hair loss. Thankfully, none of my classmates had noticed my hair loss, but because I was beginning college in the fall, I wanted to do something to make myself feel more comfortable and show my individuality. I knew that college was probably going to be the best time in my life to show that alopecia is only a part of who I am, not totally who I am. So, I made what was the probably the boldest decision of my life. I shaved my head!

I will never forget the day I shaved my head for the first time. It was on a Saturday morning, about 9am. I woke up before everyone else, and I don't know what prompted me to make the decision to shave my head. All I know is that I went outside to take a walk, and when I stopped walking, I was in front of the barbershop a few blocks up the street. I asked the barber to cut my hair off with a straight razor, and when the barber finished, I put a bandana on my head and walked back home. By the time I got home, everyone was up and moving. So, not to be subtle about it, I walked into the house, said, "BOY, it's hot outside!" and swept off the bandana. Everyone freaked out! I think I spent the entire day with everyone in the household rubbing my head and just looking – it wasn't because I was bald because everyone was used to that – rather; it was because I had willingly removed my hair instead of letting alopecia take the last few strands. The first time I shaved my head represented the first time I exerted control over my appearance and how I felt about myself, and I have tried to maintain that control since then.

Alopecia and adulthood

In the 18 years since I shaved my head for the first time, I have lived with long periods of full regrowth, and longer periods of total baldness. With AA, it is never just a patch here or there. In my case, AA generally develops very quickly into AT, and as I approach my 40s, I begin to see more symptoms of the AT becoming AU. I have smooth patches across my body, including the pubic regions, and I have lost my eyelashes cyclically. This latest period of loss, I believe, was triggered by the sudden, traumatic death of my beloved father in January 2002. At the time of his death, I was 23 years old. My father, whose calm demeanor and cool intellect were my rock during the darkest years of my childhood, was my best friend. I could talk to my father about anything, and he would listen without being judgmental, offer his advice on how to handle the situation, and trust me to make the right decision regarding the situation. As an adult, we would carpool together to work – we both worked the graveyard shift – and we had both returned to college at about the same time. At the time of his death, he was so excited about me returning to college to get another degree that it was all he talked about during the last week of his life. We read together, studied together, watched sports together, and generally enjoyed each other's company. Most important of all, he was the constant buffer between my mother and me. When her controlling tendencies and over-protectiveness pushed me to the brink of losing my temper, many times, it was his intervention that prevented all-out warfare. There were so many lessons I learned from my father, and yet so much more I will never learn from him, that I can scarcely put them all down on paper. With his loss, I felt myself beginning to drift. It took a year for my hair to fall out completely again, but by the time the first anniversary of his passing rolled around in 2003, I was once again completely bald. In the years since then, I have had very brief periods of partial regrowth, but never the total regrowth I had enjoyed in the years immediately before my father's death. In a sense, I wear my baldness as a lasting mark of my grief and sorrow at losing my best friend. The death of a parent, especially an untimely death, is not something from which any child ever recovers. I'm no exception.

Since becoming an adult, I have often found myself in the unique position of coming across former classmates who either never knew about my alopecia or were some of my biggest bullies and tormentors when we were in school. Usually, they would run into my mother or my sister and prostrate themselves with apologies for the way they treated me all those years. I have received several apologies personally, and while I accept them all graciously, I can't help but be a bit ambivalent about them as well. From my parents and my grandmother, I learned about the healing power of forgiveness alongside those lessons of right and wrong that every child learns. By the time I became an adult, I had forgiven most of the people who picked on me in my childhood as well as the adults who rejected me as a grown woman. By receiving these apologies, the door that was formerly closed became merely open again, and as an adult, it is increasingly difficult to close that door again. Perhaps, it is this repression of all the anger and sadness I felt as a child that has led me to seek out other alopecia as an adult. In all the years growing up, I never once ran into another person with AA, and people almost always assumed that I had cancer and was going through chemotherapy. I have friends, true enough, but only a handful are close enough to me to be considered true friends and confidants and/or confidantes. This select circle, none of whom are alopecia victims, all have known me both during my periods of full regrowth as well as my periods of full baldness. They have loved me unconditionally just the same. They are considered extended members of the family, and I truly cherish them.

In the years since I originally wrote my story, I have been blessed with several opportunities to share my story about alopecia through various forms of media. I have given interviews to local news stations about my experiences with alopecia. My story has been published in two books, and I maintain a blog on Alopecia World, a social networking site designed to provide resources and support for anyone suffering from alopecia areata or other forms of hair loss. I have metamorphosed from casual makeup connoisseur to full-fledged beauty junkie, and often, I provide tutorials on how to make oneself look and feel one's very best with makeup. I have traveled across the country to meet others who, like me, live with alopecia areata every day, and I can honestly say that there is truly strength in sharing an experience.

I have also become very outspoken about the need for increased education, awareness, and research into the causes of alopecia. Increased awareness is needed because, despite all the medical advances made so far and the loosening of societal boundaries regarding women and their appearance, there are still some people who view alopecia as an oddity – a walking freak show with a "strange affliction" that will do absolutely anything to make their hair grow. Nothing can be further from the truth. I, like my fellow victims alopecia, am the same red-blooded individual with hopes, dreams, emotions, and fears; just the same as anybody else. We do not want to be treated any differently than anyone else; all we want is to be accepted for who we are and not judged based solely on our physical appearance. Despite all of this, there is a greater cause for hope than ever before. With recent medical breakthroughs; most importantly, the discovery of the genetic markers that trigger hair loss in humans by famed the Columbia University geneticist, Angela Christiano, who suffers from alopecia herself, I am more hopeful than ever that a cure will be found in my lifetime. This research, combined with increased exposure in the media due to the alopecia diagnoses of celebrities such as NBA star, Charlie Villanueva; actors, Viola Davis, Sir Patrick Stewart, and Countess Vaughn; the late rap artist, Chris Kelly; and many others, brings new awareness and momentum to alopecia awareness and research as never seen before.

So, how has alopecia affected me throughout my life? Simply put, it has molded me into a shrewd, intelligent, gregarious woman, yet it has also made me a more empathetic person. I truly identify with the sufferings of others and go out of my way not to hurt the feelings of anyone with the words that I say, because having been a victim of hurtful words during the most vulnerable periods of my life, I truly would not wish such pain on my worst enemy. However, alopecia has also blessed me with amazing strength to withstand almost any crisis and made me fiercely protective of my independence. Alopecia is a double-edged sword; it alternately blesses and curses everyone whose life it touches. It changes and transforms us and presents us with a new reality. I told my story once upon a time ago when I was 11 years old. I am telling my story again, more than 20 years later, to remind the world that yes, I live with alopecia, but I am still here. I am still living, still thriving, and in spite of alopecia, I will fulfill the potential my grandmother and my parents saw years ago. I will change the world – and I will do that by telling my story to everyone, and touching everyone; one person at a time.

CHAPTER THREE

Raeshal

I was born in Charleston South Carolina on July 28, 1980, to Alice and Ray Solomon. At six months old, my parents found out that I had sickle cell after taking me to the hospital because I wouldn't stop crying. They both had the trait but didn't know it because they had never been tested. As a young girl, I was definitely a daddy's little girl and a tomboy. My father was a mechanic, so I was always underneath the car or helping him with home improvement projects around the house. My younger brother and I were always very close. We have an older sister, but she is much older, and our age gap is very obvious.

"This is my journey," a six-year-old girl whispers in her soft voice. "Daddy, Daddy, can you come here for a minute, please?" she says and whispers something in his ear so quietly no one but him can hear it. He gently wraps her up in the sheets, picks her up and puts her in the car. He quickly but cautiously drives purposely, determined to miss all the bumps. They arrive at their destination, he picks her up, walks her to the front of the church in the middle of service and lays her broken body on the altar. The six-year-old begins to pray and ask God to fix her, to take away some of the pain so she can at least breathe again. And He does exactly that. She makes a sign for her father to come, and he takes her to the hospital. Fast-forward to ten years, the little girl is now a young lady. Her sickle cell has not left her body, but she is happy to go to school pain-free. For as long as she can remember God has been her one and only true weapon against the pain that her body causes her. In times of pain, she prays pray for breath; she prays for lesser pain. She prays and asks why. She prays without tears. In times of pain, some days, weeks, and months are spent in the hospital, and you must fight depression, loneliness, and fear. She prays for peace; she prays for strength, she prays for understanding, she prays for courage, and she prays pray for mental stability.

At the age of fifteen, my mother, brother, and I moved to Nashville Tennessee. My sister was in college by then, and my dad stayed in South Carolina. My brother and I, two country kids, were like a fish out of water, but we quickly adapted to city life. Mom worked a lot, so I watched over my brother. Living in Tennessee was the first time I had to spend the night in the hospital alone. Mom couldn't do it all, besides I was sixteen years old, a teenager. I began working my first job as a server at the Waffle House; later I returned as a general manager. I graduated high school in Tennessee at the age of eighteen because I had failed the first grade in South Carolina. My teacher said I was behind in reading due to my regular absence. I didn't care, I graduated, and that's all that mattered. I started college in the fall of 1999 and graduated summer 2006. Yes, it took seven years, but who cares? I graduated; that's what counts. In those seven years, I also grieved the passing of my dad, grandma, and grandpa. I found out that I usually slowed up sometimes, but I didn't give up. Five years later, I was already a young woman, but my lungs were not working. I was in college in my twenties, walking around campus with an oxygen tank. I was sleeping with oxygen and in need of blood transfusions once a month now. I was so depressed, but I didn't want to die. I didn't have any kids. I hadn't experienced life as a normal young adult of my age. I was scared. So, I cried, and I cried. I prayed, and I prayed, "Please, God, heal my body! Take this sickle cell away from my blood and make me whole. Make me well, use me." I said this prayer over and over again for a month. Now years later, I can't remember the last time I was in the hospital for sickle cell crisis. I had the opportunity to travel all over the United States, and some other countries, too. I was now experiencing life, the abundant life Jesus talked about. However, while in college, I almost always had a full-time job and an apt. I even started my first management job in college. I also traveled to Bermuda twice and the Bahamas once. After college, I moved to Charlotte North Carolina where I got a great job working for an IT firm. I traveled and handled Human Resource duties, even purchased my first house at age twenty-six. My mom and I started taking yearly trips. After the

Human Resource job, I decided it was time for a change, and I moved to Las Vegas, Nevada, although I had been there a few times before. I loved it, but after only six months, it was time to move back to Tennessee because it was so far from family. I missed our Sunday family day dinners. I moved back into my home and became a manager of a grocery store. During all of those episodes, I still got sick a number of times. I had to leave the grocery store because it was just too physical. While managing a restaurant, I met my son's father. I took a leave from the restaurant because of a troubled pregnancy. My son had to come first, and now I only work a few hours a day, so I could be well for him. When I was pregnant with my son, and he was strong and healthy. "I'm going to be a mama," I thought to myself. At times I could work a full-time job and not be sick and not be tired. I was so happy! My son and I would spend some time at the park, doing fun things. I wanted to live a stress-free life for him. I prayed over him every day. Many people with my disease might not have the kind of fulfilling life God allowed me to have. I learned as a younger woman that it's OK to slow down when one needed to; just as long as one prayed, believed, and didn't quit.

At the age of thirty-four, my doctors are amazed at how healthy I am, and they want me to speak on a panel to doctors and nurses involved in the day-to-day care of sickle cell patients. To God Be the Glory!

CHAPTER FOUR

LaToya

What is Faith? Faith is the substance of things hoped for and the evidence of things not seen (Hebrews11:1). Faith is not contagious, neither can it be imitated; it is a personal experience.

Yes, I may be a young woman, but life has definitely afforded me enough experiences to give me gainful knowledge and respect for the quote, "We're just like tea bags, you never know how strong you really are, until you're in hot water."

So, there are some things that only your faith and prayer will carry you through and bring you out of. I pray that these next few pages inspire and enlighten you to become all that you were created for despite the obstacles set before you. God is sovereign and shows immeasurable grace by bringing His people out of trials victoriously so that He may be magnified. Obstacles, trials, and magnified are all words that can describe how my life has transitioned over the last decade. My first obstacle began in 1996, and it literally stripped me of everything I thought I had accomplished. I had to withdraw from college because of my frequent hospital admissions and surgeries of a disease that no doctor could even explain at that time. I could no longer enjoy the outdoor activities and numerous other things with my family and friends because of the chronic lung disease, known as COPD that had worsened over the years in addition to the rare bacterial infection that no one could explain at that time.

I had numerous tumors in my nasal cavity and passageway, so I couldn't smell or taste certain foods. The lists of my struggles seemed to grow longer by the day. At that time, all I heard in the church was "Press pass your pain!" But what did that really mean? Well, my translation of that was like being blindfolded, walking through an unfamiliar territory, and that was exactly how I felt at that time. Because just when things seemed like they couldn't get any worse... they would usually do.

As the years progressed and my doctors had me on a pretty steady medication regimen, the inevitable happened. I had an exacerbation that was unlike the others in the past. Now, the chronic lung disease that I suffered from was asthma, so the usual airway restrictions always made me feel like something heavy was being placed on my chest, and I would have to breathe through a straw simultaneously. No Fun!! But this felt more like I was being punched in my side, and the breath was being knocked out of me repeatedly. After the necessary tests were done, I was informed that my right lung had collapsed!! And I was headed for surgery.

Now, at this stage in my life, surgery was nothing new to me. I'd already had eight (8), one of which was the removal of sarcoma. But I sure didn't want to have another one, so I (along with the family that was there with me) did what we knew to do; I asked God to fix it. And He Did!!! The emergency room was extremely busy that night, so it was a while before doctors could come back in to "prep me" for surgery. Just enough time for us to make a connection... "All things work together for the good of them that love God..." Romans 8:28. When the doctors and nurses finally returned, they saw an amazing turnaround, took another x-ray and saw no evidence of a collapsed lung. They witnessed a miracle!!

I made a vow to God that I would forever praise him for all of the things and miracles He did in my life. So, I began ministering through mime. It not only blessed thousands, but it blessed and encouraged me every time I ministered. I know some people reading this may wonder, "How can she dance when she has such an extensive medical/breathing condition?" I don't have any real fancy answer to that one, all I know is, God has kept me, and He is still keeping me! And you'll understand when I'm done explaining my next trial.

As always, I give my all when I am asked or invited to minister because of the promise I made to God. So, I did just that, and after the dance was over, I ended up in the emergency department again. This time, it was worse than before. At one point, I stopped breathing and was put on a ventilator for two days. I found out later that the attending doctors didn't expect me to make it out of the hospital alive. This was by far the scariest experience ever to date. Since then, my health has improved dramatically. I haven't had any ICU admissions or ER visits. Although I am on a strict medication regimen of nineteen prescriptions daily and steroid-dependent, I, along with my physicians, am working diligently to minimize my medication intake permanently. When I mentioned that God would be magnified, that's a very true statement. Through all of those obstacles and trials, God still opened doors. I graduated from college with honors, I have four wonderful children, and a great husband who makes provision for me to live my dream every day.

I may be struggling with an illness, but my illness certainly doesn't have me. It has always been my prayer to never look like what I'm going through... Many Blessings!

CHAPTER FIVE

———~~———

Aretha

A Kiss from God…

"This is a woman thing, take as many pills as you need." This was the doctor's response to the excruciating pain I endured every month during my cycle. By this time, I was a teenager, and I was consistently popping painkillers like candy, 4 and 5 at times, but they would not stay down. I had **endometriosis,** and it was taking over my life. It started when I was twelve (12) years old and slowly began to dominate my life. It went from pain determined as "normal" to being totally unbearable. Along with the pain came other side effects that challenged any kind of normality. For the first 3 to 4 days of my cycle, I could not stand the smell of food. I would run from the aroma and find myself in the bathroom to regurgitate. I could not lie on the bed because its soft surface would amplify my pains. My body was so sensitive that when lying on the floor, I could feel any approaching footsteps, which would always cause my stomach to shake. I remember feeling like a vicious animal had its sharp teeth stuck on the side of my stomach. After a while, I got used to the idea that I would have to deal with the pain indefinitely, after all, the doctor said: "This is normal."

Finally, after fifteen 15 plus years, I had enough! I was bent over, crying out in pain to the Lord, "It's too much! I am tired of this!" My official meltdown had finally happened. After my spirit had calmed, I heard the Lord say, "Why don't you ask me for healing?" I paused in silence. It's like I woke up. In essence, I did. Immediately, I began to have a conversation with myself. "Why haven't you asked for healing?" I definitely believed in healings. In those few minutes, I realized I bought into the doctor's gospel instead of God who loved me. I responded to the Lord's request. "God, will you heal me?" With a loving response, He said, "Yes, I will."

It was a Bible study night, and despite the pain, I made it. The co-pastor asked if there was anyone that needed prayer. I quickly responded and made my request for the first time: "I want prayer to be healed." The co-pastor called for assistance from a friend of mine that had not too long joined our faith community. We prayed in agreement. I was asked after the prayer, "Are you still in pain?" … "Yes," I responded. I was asked again. I felt because of the second request, I must have given the wrong answer, so I said, "No" as a faith statement though I still felt the pain. I went home that night a little discouraged, but I had heard a Word from God that He would heal me. I grabbed my glass of water and pills that I usually kept by the bed for the pain that normally awakened me, and I went to sleep, believing that someday, I would have the manifestation of my healing. At 4:00 am, I was awakened. The house was quiet. My roommate was a nurse. She regularly worked the 3rd shift. She was not home at the time. All I could hear was the clock. I lay there and took a quick assessment of my body. No pain, no pain, no pain! Then all of a sudden, I felt two hands enter my womb. "What is happening?" I asked to myself. There was no fear; there was such peace. I felt these hands go into my womb gently and turn it. I said out loud, "Lord, is that you?" He answered me by putting the finishing touches on my miracle. He turned my womb, with a few adjustments, and like a vacuum, sucked it into the right position. I could hear my womb lock in place. Yes, I had endometriosis but what I did not know was that my womb was tilted, too. The Great Physician did great work on me! I lay there with peace flooding my soul! The old hymn, "He Touched Me" came to mind.

"He touched me, Oh He touched me

Oh what joy that floods my soul

Something happened

And now, I know

He touched me

And made me whole."

I lay there with tears streaming down my face, consumed in the presence of God. "What just happened?" Without delay, I got up, no pain, showered, no pain, went to work, no pain, and I shared what happened to me with a friend who had been having female complications. As I shared my encounter, she got healed!!

Several years later, I married and was pregnant. I was reminded of the Lord's promise. "Proof of your healing will be that you will have a son." I refused to have an ultrasound to determine the gender of our child. To me, it was just a stand of faith in what the Lord had spoken. It was time for delivery and with only one good push, came a beautiful baby boy!

God is so faithful to His Word! The friend that agreed in prayer that day over my healing became my husband and the father of our miracle child, Timothy Stephen, who is regarded with great affection. I call him my KFG, "Kiss from God." He is the constant reminder of the love of the Father and the touch that healed me.

May you have lots of Kisses from the Father. Amen!

CHAPTER SIX

———— ∞ ————

Reality

Now that you've heard testimonies and shared in the journey of women like yourself (or know of someone going through similar struggles) be inspired to live and help others live their lives beyond any medical condition. It was my desire to include the stories of victorious women that did extraordinary things. Women of different cultures were sought out to tell of their experiences so prayerfully. This book will be the first of many. It is my belief that whatever challenges we face, that is what changes us and gives us the opportunity to speak into someone else' life. Never feel as though you have to prove anything or that you owe anyone, accept God who created you. When you please the creator by being grateful, thankful, and appreciative for life given to you, watch how He will use you to make a difference in the world. To God, we give praise and honor for all He has done. Your circumstance may not change overnight, but you will begin to see things manifest in yourself as you draw closer to Jesus Christ by studying, believing and acting upon His word through faith, hope, and love. Know Him for yourself! I can personally say I have never seen the righteous forsaken or God's seed, His children, those Jesus died for, beg bread. "For God so loved the world that he gave his only begotten son that whosoever believes in him should not perish but shall have life everlasting."

Before I leave you, I would like to share just one more story of a young lady who lived in unbearable pain. She spent years bleeding and crying behind closed doors; she experienced surgeries, married and then went through a horrendous miscarriage of her first child. The couple was so young with great expectations, but with this devastation, they found it impossible to maintain their marriage, and so, divorced.

More surgeries were necessary because of the endometriosis, but in spite of the struggle and suggestion of hysterectomy by doctors, she refused to abort her faith. After a few years, she remarried and was blessed to birth her own child, a son by the name of Samuel. May I introduce you to Hannah, my third child, my daughter, born with a declared promise and a grandma's wit. Stay tuned for our next edition of God's Elect Ladies and hear more about the miraculous power of God.

As a preacher trying to wrap up a message of hope, I wondered why I could not move forward in the publishing of this book, but God was faithful to let me know you're not quite done. God's Elect Ladies touches the silent as well as the vocal women who live their lives in the shadow, who have hushed their truths, believing they live in hopeless situations. What I have shared is worth talking about, it's real. The names of these women have been withheld because it could be you or me. Some women have lived, and others are living a life of hurt and shame. We could have titled this chapter Abandoned, Hurt, Confused, Abused and many other words that had come to mind. It is like an emotional roller coaster strapped in verbalism and physical pain but not because of physical sickness or disease but a terminal emotional illness.

Strippers, prostitutes, adulteresses, drug addicts, homosexuals, and others are often stereotyped because of what we see from the surface of a person. However, I have learned the person we see is not always who they are but who they have become; born out of an evil experience. We should not be fooled by these titles because some of the deepest secrets are well kept and managed even among the elites and the well-dressed. Many people appear to have it together with saintly mannerism, but their appearance is far from the truth. Their history has been tainted by molestation, painful beatings and fear of being sold through sex trafficking. Some have been abused from childhood to adulthood and contaminated by the spirit of lust. It does not matter that life's situations are stuffed in closets, attics or hidden in the dungeon of a wounded soul, abuse makes little girls afraid and anesthetizes young ladies. This is the reason for which most women drink until they get drunk, smoke until they get high, take drugs until they pass-out, and advertise their bodies. It is to cover a silent sickness. It brings confusion, abortions, abandonment, and suicide.

Long-term abuse gradually becomes normal and it affects the behavior of its victims. Image being verbally, physically, sexually, and emotionally abused until it becomes the norm. So many of our beautiful sisters seeking affirmation beautify their lips, enlarge their boobs, thicken their booties and mark themselves with tattoos with the hope to find love and fill the empty void. Ethnicity, age social status and education status do not shield women from abuse, and the effect is the same. The good news is, Jesus loves each of us as we are. And just as He healed the woman with the issue of blood and the Syro-Phoenician woman's daughter that was possessed and freed her from spiritual bondage, so will He do the same today. The question is, "Do you want to be healed?" God so loved the world that He included Rahab the prostitute, Mary Magdalene, and many others who were twisted and tangled in Satan's web in His redemptive mission. There's no barrier with Jesus. Jesus' love is illustrated in each of us by reaching, teaching, and loving one another. Remember this, the next time you see a sister in the red-light district painted up for attention or abandoning her children for a high, she is terminally ill and needs as much help as any physically ill woman.

We are God's Elect Women, strong and courageous, and we love the sisters and daughters of God. We open our hearts, our doors, and opportunities for hope! If you have a story or testimony that will make a difference in someone's life, we invite you to share it and be a blessing.